MW01232266

The first step in losing weight and creating a life change is to schedule an initial consultation (conducted in-person or over the phone) with our dedicated and compassionate team. This is a $25 value, but as a reader of this book, you pay nothing when you mention code **PHDlife**.

During this meeting, we will:

- Learn about your story, health history and goals.

- Explain how PHD works uniquely for you.

- Answer all of your questions.

At the end of our time together, you will:

- Know if PHD is a good fit for you.

- Understand why you've experienced weight gain and what your Optimal Weight is.

- Know the length and cost of your customized program and will be able to get started immediately if you choose.

- Have peace of mind knowing that you have the science, support, and accountability pieces in place to allow for successful weight loss once and for all.

To schedule:

Call 1-800-674-8991 and choose the option that is most convenient to you!

5 STEPS TO RESET THE SCALE

Discover Why Weight Gain Is Not Your Fault and How to Take the Weight Off for Good

Dr. Ashley Lucas, RD

PhD Nutritionist and Registered Dietitian

PUBLISHED BY
PHD Advanced Nutrition, LLC
1833 Hendersonville Rd.
Asheville, NC 28803
828.552.3333

Copyright © 2022

All rights reserved. Without limiting the rights under copyright reserved above, no part of this book may be reproduced, stored or introduced into a retrieval system, or transmitted, in any form or by any means (electronic, mechanical, photocopying, recording or otherwise), without the prior written permission of both the copyright owner and the publisher.

072222

DISCLAIMER:

This book contains the opinions and ideas of the author. The purpose of this book is to provide you with helpful information about weight loss and good health. This book should not be used to diagnose or treat any medical condition. Careful attention has been paid to ensure the accuracy of the information, but the author cannot assume responsibility for the validity or consequences of its use. This information is not intended to diagnose or treat any disease. The material in this book is for informational purposes only. As each individual situation is unique, the author disclaims responsibility for any adverse effects that may result from the use or application of the information contained in this book. Any use of the information found in this book is the sole responsibility of the reader. Any suggestions found in this book are to be followed only under the supervision of a medical doctor.

CONTENTS

Part 4—The Path Forward

Part 5—References

DEDICATION

To my husband, Doug, and my three kids, Dash, Gage and Pemma. For their unconditional support of my crazy dreams and my fighter jet mentality, which I know can be exhausting at times. ☺

To the amazing PHD team for always showing up to serve others and their burning desire to help people live the best life possible.

To every single PHD client for stepping up, doing the work, and having the courage, dedication, and commitment to being a positive force for good in their own lives and those around them.

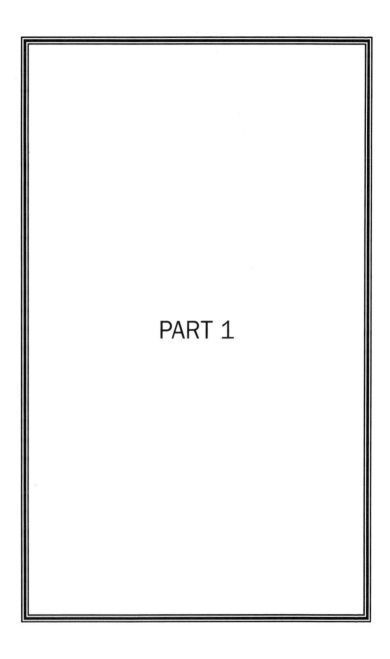

PART 1

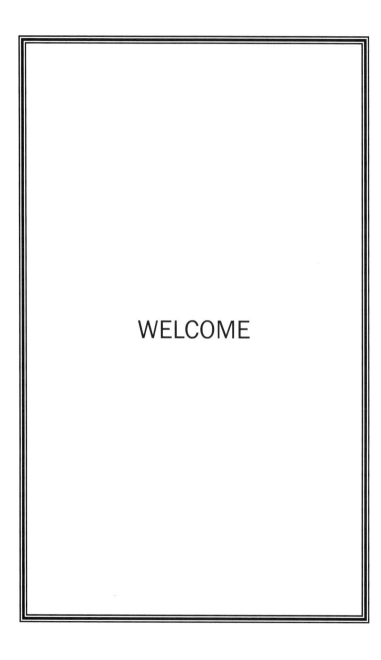

WELCOME

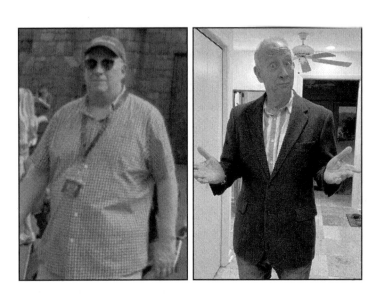

Mike Gallagher Before & After (down 44 lbs.)

FOREWORD

As a national radio host, I'm often asked to endorse products and services. For years, I've been approached by various weight loss companies and programs. Despite having a lifelong weight challenge, I've always resisted doing an on-air endorsement in this category.

Since I've tried everything—counting points, fasting, raw food, you name it—I wasn't really confident in sharing a weight loss attempt on-air. That is, until PHD Weight Loss and Nutrition came into my life.

I had been hearing about Dr. Ashley Lucas and her innovative, successful program for some time. Every friend who tried PHD Weight Loss experienced dramatic and joyful weight loss. All of them raved about PHD. *"I'm never hungry,"* they'd say. *"I'm eating better than ever. I've never felt this good in my life."*

When one of my friends lost over 100 pounds on PHD Weight Loss—and swore it was one of the easiest things he'd ever done—I had to try it.

After several months, I'm now 44 pounds lighter than when I began. And everything my friends told me was correct: I never experience hunger pangs, I'm eating so much healthier than I ever had been. (Who knew that I would actually start loving veggies?) And the weight keeps dropping off, week after week. I love the PHD foods! (If Heaven doesn't have their peanut butter bar, I'm not entirely sure I wanna go!)

And I am so grateful for the guidance I get from Rachel, my coach. I look forward to our weekly calls as she gives me all kinds of tips and food suggestions and inspiration.

For me, the most important thing about the PHD Weight Loss journey is to finally lose that stubborn, visceral belly fat that I've carried around for most of my adult life. Well, I'm about 12 pounds away from my goal, my "Optimal Weight." And there is simply no doubt in my mind that I will get there soon.

Starting this plan is the smartest thing I've done in many, many years. And now I am proud to enthusiastically and officially endorse PHD Weight Loss and Nutrition on my radio show.

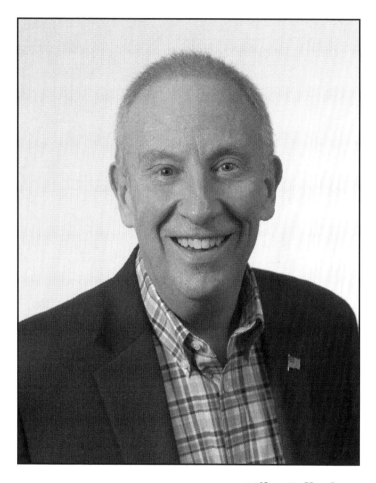

—**Mike Gallagher**
Salem Radio Network
Tampa, Florida & New York City, New York

"My experience with PHD has been a lifesaving one. It's hard to put it in words how grateful I am to this program. A year ago, before I found PHD, I was in a place of complacency that I would never be the person I used to be. I'm so glad I had a life-altering moment of fear and desperation and picked up the phone and called PHD."

—PHD Client, Janet

WHO SHOULD READ
THIS BOOK?

Collapsing time. One of our very most precious gifts in life is time. It goes by so fast, and I personally never feel that I have enough of it. I bet you feel similarly. One of my primary goals in all of my work is to help people collapse time: to drop weight faster, more effectively, more efficiently, and sustainably so they can go on living a better life, a life that they deserve and desire, as quickly and successfully as possible.

Thus, although I wrote this book to be read in about an hour, I definitely don't want to waste your time here if this content is not for you. Please take a few minutes and read this entire section to see if *5 Steps to Reset the Scale* is a smart investment of your energy and focus. I wrote this short book for four reasons:

1. To dispel the 3 most common weight loss myths that ultimately lead to weight loss failure and frustrations so that you can avoid falling into the trap.

2. To explain why weight gain really isn't your fault and why it is much more complicated than calories in and calories out.

3. To provide 5 clear steps to lose weight and successfully maintain it for the long-term.

4. To invite you to connect with me so we can determine if working with PHD Weight Loss and implementing the **Reset the Scale Method**™ is right for you.

While just about any person struggling with weight issues can benefit from working with PHD Weight Loss, I wrote *5 Steps to Reset the Scale* for 5 main groups of people who I have seen benefit the most from my *Reset the Scale Method.*

Over the last 10 years of practice, I have seen each of these groups of individuals lose weight so effectively and in such a sustainable manner that I feel I have a moral obligation to share the message with as many of these people as possible.

These people I speak of are:

1. Men, 45+ years old, who were once athletes (think collegiate football, basketball, baseball players, runners, etc.).

2. Busy women and moms with kids.
3. High-performing business professionals and executives.
4. Those who have tried everything with no success.
5. Those with a genetic predisposition toward overweight and obesity. (You gain weight easily; your parents struggled and so have you, for most of your life.)

These 5 groups of people have unique needs that make weight loss a bit more difficult yet for whom I have mastered the system.

Finally, *5 Steps to Reset the Scale*, was written for the person who agrees with these seven beliefs:

1. Time is the most precious gift in your life, therefore, getting help and losing weight the right way through a natural, healthy, effective and efficient weight loss approach is worth an investment of your energy and money.
2. Health is the most valuable thing in your life; you take your health seriously and realize it is more important than anything on your "to do" list.
3. It's worth investing in yourself to feel better, live better, have deeper personal relationships, more confidence, and create lasting

7

and sustainable positive changes in your life and those around you.

4.   Accountability and support is key to successful weight loss and weight loss maintenance.

5.   It's better to be coached and guided on how to drop weight successfully rather than fumbling along attempting to do it on our own, racking up one failed attempt after another.

6.   Weight loss and then maintaining it is just too complicated to do on your own, and getting a team of experts, real-live-people, to support you would be helpful. You value professional advice.

7.   Working with PHD Weight Loss is the key to dropping weight efficiently and painlessly.

If you have experienced weight loss failures in the past and/or if you are simply at a threshold where you know you *must* make a change and lose weight once and for all, I wrote this book for you. So please keep reading, and most of all, know there is hope for simple long-term weight loss success!

MY PROMISE TO YOU

I promise to make *5 Steps to Reset the Scale* a valuable use of your time and attention. This book is purposely short. I want you to be able to read and understand it quickly and easily. These days everyone and their brother professes to be a nutrition expert. There are so many misconceptions, incorrect information, myths and fad diets associated with weight loss available on the internet, which is one of the reasons why I wrote this book.

After helping thousands of people nationwide over the last decade successfully drop weight painlessly and sustainably, I want you to know that there is hope and that you too can do the same with the right tools, guidance and support in place.

I realize what you are about to read may initially be really frustrating to you as you come to understand that the majority of what you've been told, even by your doctor, about weight loss has been wrong. But, understanding the truth about WHY weight gain happens in the first place is the key to being able to take it off.

I am sharing this with you, along with the steps required to lose the weight for good (which might sound a bit unconventional), with the hope that you can finally be liberated from the suffering associated with carrying around unwanted excess fat weight.

I want you to know you CAN lose weight for the rest of your life simply because you want to.

Over the course of the next hour or so, I will:

- Help you understand why weight gain isn't your fault.

- Explain to you why weight regain happens.

- Break apart 3 common weight loss myths so you can avoid the traps.

- Teach you what the best fuel is for your body to drop weight and maintain it.

- Help you understand the mindset shift required for weight loss.

- Explain how, for many, weight loss is an addiction recovery process.

- Help you understand what's needed for long-term weight loss maintenance.

Every week I hear from clients how PHD Weight Loss and the *Reset the Scale Method* has transformed their life. They exclaim that they never imagined weight loss would be so simple, feel so good, be so satisfying and taste good all at the same time!

What I share here may be unfamiliar and unconventional, but I have good news. If you want to drop weight, break the ties with the foods you say you love that don't love you back, and move on with a vibrant life, you are reading the right book. I take your health and overall well-being very seriously. On behalf of our entire team, we live and breathe your ultimate success.

"*PHD Weight Loss is so much more than losing weight. It's about total life transformation. It's about finding your authentic self underneath the weighted cloak. It's about stepping out and living the life you have always dreamt of. It's about looking at yourself in the mirror and loving that person. It's total life transformation, and you're worth it!*"

—PHD Client, Kim

INTRODUCTION

Since you're reading these words, I'm assuming you're OK with what I've shared so far and you are ready to join me in what I hope is an eye-opening and rewarding 60 minutes as I share with you why weight loss isn't your fault and what to do about it.

I vividly remember sitting with a client in my office and her bursting out into tears when I told her that weight loss is more complicated than calories in and out. She proceeded to tell me that the amount of food she ate simply didn't account for the amount of excess fat weight (about 70 lbs.) that she was carrying. I told her I believed her, and with tears streaming down her face, she stood up and gave me a hug.

Her doctor told her that losing weight was simple: She just needed to eat less and get out and move more. But she already only ate 1200 calories, was starving all the time, and her knees ached from the inflammation and excess force pushed through her joints caused by the weight gain.

I told her that she should be able to drop weight without being hungry and that the first step to successful weight loss isn't through eating less and moving more.

She sat in disbelief, frustrated at the suffering she had experienced for over a decade while trying to lose weight through methods she had been told worked yet didn't work for her. She thought the problem was her, that she was simply a failure, and that there was no hope.

Tammy lost 70 lbs. in 28 weeks with PHD Weight Loss. Three years later, Tammy is maintaining her 70 lbs. weight loss; she's hiking, riding her horse, confident and isn't even hungry.

You see, counting calories to achieve long-term weight loss success is a bogus strategy. You are much more complicated than a simple equation or machine that has no metabolic energy needs, emotions, or day -to-day influences. Your body is not regulated by calorie sensors.

A jaw dropping statistic shows us that 95% of diets we do on our own fail. The deal is, we can't all be failures, and although we might not all be mathematical wizards, the ins and outs oftentimes just don't add up!

I'm here to tell you that weight gain isn't your fault, and the reason why you've dropped weight in the past only to regain it has nothing to do with your personality or willpower.

I'm going to share a little secret with you (well, actually, quite a few throughout this book), but to start: ***You are not a failure.*** Rather, it's the antiquated methodologies that you have tried previously that have failed you.

Before reading on, I feel it's important for you to understand that I believe in challenging the standard ways of thinking when it comes to nutrition and weight loss. Therefore, thinking and acting differently are at the core of everything we do at PHD Weight Loss, including our philosophies, our *Reset the Scale Method* and our team culture.

Throughout this book, you'll notice evidence-based concepts that haven't yet been popularized in the "industry" of weight management. I believe this is the case because these concepts support the individual's well-being (i.e., YOU) and not money-making corporations.

I am extremely pleased to be able to offer you *5 Steps to Reset the Scale*. Through this book, my mission is to create positive change in your life. I strive to empower you to step up, take action, and find the results you desire and deserve.

My goal is to help you let go of not only excess weight but also the emotions of shame, fear, guilt and unworthiness that are often tied to it. Additionally, it's important to understand that change and up-leveling yourself in any way takes commitment and determination.

You have the power to create change within yourself. All you need is a strong desire, met with the **right** action, and unwavering persistence—that's when the magic happens! My hope is that we can inspire one another to use past failures as the impetus for future success and hold each other accountable to be better than we were yesterday.

I understand weight loss can be overwhelming and scary, but it doesn't have to be that way. Although I know this book will fall short of providing you with the answers to all of your questions, it is my aim that within the subsequent pages, you will find valuable guidance, comfort in knowing that you are not alone on your journey, and that weight loss for life is indeed possible.

3 COMMON
WEIGHT LOSS MYTHS

Before I share the 5 steps, I want to dispel 3 common weight loss myths. When you're counting calories and have a consistent exercise regimen, you expect to see immediate, strong results. But, sometimes, it doesn't happen that way. That's because there are scientific explanations as to why weight loss is incredibly difficult and nearly impossible for some people without the right resources.

Much of what we know about dieting and exercise does not address human variables, as I mentioned earlier, such as environmental, genetic, and other factors that contribute to how we metabolize food. There are many reasons why the scale might not be budging as you think it should.

When you're trying to lose weight and it doesn't seem to be working, it has a lot to do with your metabolic state and what you've been through.

For example, if you're a Type 2 diabetic, your metabolism is significantly different than someone who has 20–30 pounds to drop and has no underlying medical conditions. At PHD, we look at each client and have to ask, "*What happened in this person's life that shifted how their mind or body is tolerating food?*"

Some people are naturally lean and their metabolism very tolerant, so they can eat and exercise and their bodies burn the calories easily. But that's not usually the story. The secret to successful weight loss is understanding that it's not just about science or what and when you eat; it's also about how you're thinking and feeling. Successful weight loss requires a holistic approach that tackles the mind and body in an unconventional way.

Let's talk about three common beliefs that we know **don't work** for weight loss:

MYTH #1: EXERCISE

Exercise is an awesome wellness tool that is important to maintaining a healthy lifestyle, but it's not an effective weight loss tool for most people. When you try to drop weight through exercise alone, you may experience the opposite effect.

You would need to cycle 1,000 miles or run 350 miles just to burn 10 lbs. of fat! The goal is to move because you love it. Once you improve your health and drop excess weight, your desire to move will naturally increase as you experience less pain and fatigue.

My husband, an orthopedic foot and ankle surgeon, likes to tell me that every pound of excess fat we carry on our frames, equates to 8 extra lbs. of force pushing through the ankle and 6 lbs. through the knees.

Every pound of excess fat you carry in your belly, specifically, equates to 4–5 lbs. of force pulling off your spine. If you're carrying 50 lbs. of excess fat weight, this equates to 400 lbs. of force through your ankles with each step!

My husband sees one patient after another about foot pain due to trying to exercise the weight off. His advice for these patients time and time again is to drop the weight first; reduce the amount of force pushing through those fragile joints, then think about exercise.

As much as we would like to believe it, our bodies aren't as simple as a mathematical equation. I'm not saying we defy Newton's Laws of Thermodynamics, but many issues factor into why the scale tracks up or down.

Here are some key factors to consider:

1. *What* are you eating?
2. *When* are you eating?
3. *What* is your environment and emotional state?

MYTH #2: CALORIE RESTRICTION

Severe caloric restriction is not a sustainable weight loss tool. When calories are too restricted, the metabolism slows and may not normalize over time (Johannsen, 2012). Research shows that calorie deprivation is also more likely to lead to anxiety and depression (Keys, 1950). This method might allow for a short-term weight decrease, but weight regain is very likely.

On another note, against severe calorie restriction, four tightly controlled inpatient studies compared calories consumed to calories burned. If you did the math, you would estimate that every participant should drop 10 lbs. when considering their "ins and outs." Guess what? No one did! The average person shed 7 lbs. whereas many of the participants dropped only 2–3 lbs. (Bouchard et al., 1994; Volek & Phinney, 2012; Woo et al., 1982).

MYTH #3: EATING EVERYTHING IN MODERATION & WILLPOWER

Obesity or being overweight is not a personality flaw. It's not due to lack of willpower or discipline (Taubes, 2010). Eating in moderation when many of us are addicted to food and carrying around active belly fat (see Chapter 2) leads straight to repetitive weight loss failure and frustration. Weight gain is not your fault, but it is a metabolic scenario that you can overcome.

Even though dropping the weight and maintaining it is a complicated process, ultimately, success can be broken down into 5 main steps. I am going to discuss each one in the following chapters. The 5 main steps are:

1. Fully collapsing the hungry, active fat mass that keeps you fat.

2. Understanding your metabolism and what/when you need to eat to support it.

3. Recognizing that 80% of weight loss is mental, emotional, habit, and behavior; mindset must be tackled.

4. Realizing that weight loss is an addiction recovery process for a lot of people. Dropping weight is a process of letting go.

5. Comprehending the reality that maintenance is a life-long practice that only works if you work it.

More important than any of these 5 steps is accepting the fact that outside support for success is necessary 95% of the time. Don't feel guilty or shameful. Just take action!

People don't fail diets;
diets fail people.

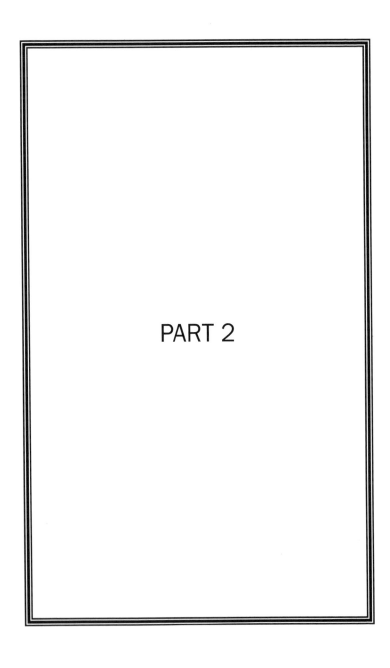

PART 2

5 STEPS TO
RESET THE SCALE

"*Now that I have lost sixty pounds with PHD Weight Loss, I feel better. I do not become winded doing simple tasks, and I am able to exercise more than twice as much as I used to be able to and still have energy to enjoy life. Food does not have the emotional hold over me that it once did. I enjoy looking and feeling more like my younger self!*"

—PHD Client, Sherry

FULLY COLLAPSE YOUR EXCESS FAT MASS & FIND YOUR OPTIMAL WEIGHT

With each passing day of our lives, our bodies change. It happens before our eyes. We look in the mirror or see a photo of ourselves, our jaw drops, and we stare in disbelief. *"Who is THAT person? It sure as heck isn't me!"*, we say to ourselves as we put on a baggier shirt and our elastic waistband pants.

Well, as sure as our outward appearance might change, our "insides" change right alongside them. When I talk with people on the topic of weight gain, they will commonly say that they don't eat any differently than they did in the past. Or they say they eat well and maintain an active lifestyle, however, regardless of their calories in and out, they continue to gain weight.

PHD Client, Sarah

When I met with Sarah, a PHD client, she said she decided to make a life change to get back to the healthy self she remembered prior to having three babies. She had tried to lose weight off-and on over the last 10 years but was never able to lose more than 10–15 pounds and would gain it back over the next year or so.

With menopause hitting, it made losing even the 10–15 pounds almost impossible. It was frustrating, and she felt like a failure. She hated the way she felt in her clothes. Her confidence suffered, and so did her sex life. She felt tired a lot and unable to do the things she used to do with ease.

She was simply over feeling terrible day in and day out. She specifically said she wanted her kids to look at her like she was someone they were proud of and wanted her husband to be attracted to her again. She felt she was not the person he married. She said while looking back, *"I know he still loved me, but I guess I just didn't love myself anymore. I had let myself go and wasn't proud of that."*

PHD Client, Bill

Bill, a 55-year-old PHD client, came in to see us with about 70 lbs. to drop. He carried the majority of his weight in his belly, chest, and throat area. As a result, he suffered from heartburn, sleep apnea, hormonal imbalance (low testosterone and high estrogen), and high blood pressure. He also feared a diagnosis of Type 2 diabetes coming down the pipeline any day.

He felt addicted to food. "Food is my drug of choice," he would tell me. His weight started piling on in his 30s when he took on a stressful job and was trying to survive in an unhappy marriage. When we spoke, he was divorced but embarrassed to start dating.

He wanted to return to the activities he did in his 20s but couldn't do anymore because of fatigue, pain, and an honest lack of physical ability to do what he loved. He felt his quality of life wasn't where he ever imagined it would be. He was about to retire and wanted to enjoy his "freedom" but couldn't actually do anything, at least in the way he wanted to do it.

Triggers

As we travel through our lives, we experience different stressors, which I like to think of as *triggers*. These triggers, which vary from one person to the next, change the way that we tolerate our food.

Examples of common triggers are puberty, major lifestyle changes, stressors (jobs, relationships, etc.), pregnancy, menopause, injury, general aging, and for those of us who are really lucky, our own birth (in other words, a heavy genetic predisposition).

If we look at Sarah's situation, we can see quite a few triggers layered on top of one another: pregnancy, menopause, major lifestyle changes, and likely more that we don't know about. The same is true of Bill. He experienced significant stressful triggers (job, marriage, and divorce) that shifted his metabolic tolerance causing him to no longer tolerate the types of foods and/or amounts of food he used to eat.

Like Sarah and Bill, your body also changes in response to such triggers.

For example, your hair might fall out, your nails might become brittle, or you might develop acne. Following a trigger, you may continue to eat the same way that you ate in the past. These eating habits may once have enabled you to maintain a healthy weight, yet these same habits now result in weight gain.

This often causes confusion, and rightly so, because it doesn't make sense, especially when we consider the "calorie in and out" paradigm that we've been told for so long governs our weight. Well, weight gain and loss aren't so simple.

It's not that your metabolism is "bad" now or that you've done something wrong. It just means that your body has changed. These triggers have altered your metabolism and have created a shift in how you tolerate food and drink of the past; what may have worked before no longer does.

Following the onset of these triggers and the resulting shift in your metabolic tolerance, you'll notice that your body shape begins to change as you start to accumulate fat primarily in the belly. This belly fat, known as *visceral fat*, is the primary culprit for ease of continued fat storage once weight gain has started. This deep, gel-like fat packs in your belly area, fills up your organs, squeezes them tight, and makes your liver look like a Kobe beef steak (medically termed fatty liver).

It is different from the rest of the fat in your body because you can't melt, laser, suck, freeze, or sculpt it away. This special fat grows blood vessels, has an oxygen supply, and secretes toxic hormones.

What you have actually accumulated in your belly is really metabolically active tissue. This fat mass has its own agenda—a mind of its own—and it is completely unregulated. All that this tissue wants to do is continue to grow as fast as possible, much like a tumor does. All of the hormones it secretes in your body are intended to encourage its continued growth. This fat is like an entity in and of itself. It has urges, demands, desires, and cravings.

The more fat mass that you have, the more addictions to food you have. This fat mass slows your metabolism, makes you hungry, triggers cravings, and makes you "lazy." Your body simply doesn't want to move and only wants to store more fat.

At this point in your weight gain, your signals of hunger and fullness are out of whack, and you don't know up from down in terms of what your body is telling you to eat or not eat.

This visceral, tumor-like fat also secretes significant inflammatory hormones. Interleukin-6, a cytokine which is a hormone-like signaling molecule, is the main culprit, which is linked to increased cancer, heart disease risk and more (Mohamed-Ali et al., 1997).

This is also one of the reasons why overweight and obese individuals are at higher risk of developing severe COVID-19. The virus itself causes a release of interleukin-6 and additionally triggers the visceral (belly) fat cells to substantially increase their levels of interleukin-6 secretions. Together with the already high baseline level of inflammation and now with the additional secretions of interleukin-6 during the infection, a cytokine storm may ensue.

This ultimately results in so much inflammation that in many cases, the overweight and obese body can't tolerate the load and severe infection results (Mehta & Fajgenbaum, 2021; Silverio et al., 2021).

Visceral belly fat also secretes hormones that lower testosterone in men and increases the risk of estrogen-dependent breast cancer in women. This fat is a beast and may be the culprit for why you've dropped weight in the past only to regain it.

Remember Sarah's story of dropping 10–15 pounds only to regain it? This wasn't due to a flaw in her willpower, it's the visceral fat effect. She still had ample visceral fat remaining, working against her, secreting hormones that disrupted her metabolism and physiology.

And Bill? This is why he had low testosterone and higher estrogen levels. If you're a man and carry belly fat, you're likely right there with him. Carrying weight in the belly will disrupt your hormones. And as you continue to gain more fat, it will accumulate heavily in the belly, chest, and throat area, indicative of higher estrogen levels and putting you at risk for high blood pressure, sleep apnea, and heart attack, just like Bill.

To minimize the risk of weight regain and be able to maintain your weight loss, you must let go of all of the visceral fat that is causing this metabolic slowing. An analogy I like to use is that of a weed. If you only chop the top off of a weed and leave the root, it will only grow back again.

You must also understand that dropping weight and successfully maintaining it requires a different way of eating from the past *for the rest of your life.* Fortunately, these changes should feel and look outstanding!

When Sarah first began adjusting her way of eating, she noticed positive changes in the first few days. Her heartburn went away, and she wasn't hungry all the time. She slept better, and she lost 8 pounds in the first week!

She told me she didn't expect to feel so good overall while losing the weight. Like many of our clients' initial expectations, she thought she would be hungry and miserable during the process. However, within 3 weeks of starting her program, she said she could not recall a time when she had felt better! Even while dropping weight each week, she felt great and had more energy. She looked like herself again and felt so much better in every way.

Bill dropped 70 lbs., normalized his hormones, reversed his high blood pressure, and said goodbye to the potential of diabetes. He broke through the chains of food addiction, and today you can find him dating, enjoying his retirement, and hiking the trails in the high-altitude terrain of Colorado.

If you have tried to drop weight in the past only to regain it, do not think of yourself as a failure. Recognize your triggers, accept the fact that you must make a change to fully get rid of the hungry/active fat mass, dig out the root, and adjust the way that you eat to support your optimal health for the long term.

"I haven't been this healthy, or at this weight, since high school. I was stuck in a spiral of guilt, shame, and emotional eating, and PHD came along and showed me positivity, a joyful journey, and how to let go—literally and figuratively. I have learned to trust my body, and to eat to live, not live to eat! I have my life back. Thank you, PHD!"

—PHD Client, Tracey

FOCUS ON THE RIGHT FUEL

Current statistics show that 75% of the American population is overweight, and 42% are obese. A whopping 88% of us are metabolically unwell, leaving only 12% of Americans on the road to health (Hales et al., 2020; Hyman, 2016). These statistics simply demonstrate that proposed conventional solutions to overcoming weight gain and illness don't work for the majority of us.

We are finding that metabolic variability, or in other words, teaching the body how to burn fat for fuel, allows many of us to experience better health and wellness.

To achieve this metabolic shift, in general, we need to be aware of our carbohydrate tolerance and eat within it, enjoy a moderate amount of protein, and increase our consumption of dietary fat. While eating more dietary fat might seem counterintuitive, research shows and clinical evidence supports that eating plenty of healthy fat during weight loss helps the body burn fat more efficiently and prevents damage to your metabolism.

Also, the reason why carbohydrate reduction is effective in treating overweight, obesity, and myriad other health conditions is because carbs have the most profound effect on how we metabolize other nutrients and how our body regulates fat metabolism.

If you've suffered from weight issues (particularly if your excess fat stores surround your stomach), you are likely intolerant of carbohydrates on some level; your body has a dysfunctional response following carbohydrate consumption. This is not your fault; it's simply how your body responds to various nutrients.

Becoming aware of your carbohydrate intake doesn't necessarily mean you have to eliminate them completely. Carbs aren't evil! The *Reset the Scale Method* doesn't require you to follow a defined dietary protocol (e.g., Ketogenic, Atkins®, Whole 30, etc.). What we do instead is investigate your carbohydrate tolerance level and eat to support what your unique body can tolerate.

So, what should you eat?

For the purpose of this book, we are going to focus on just the first half of the day, starting with breakfast. Breakfast has been touted as the most important meal of the day. Spoiler alert—research shows this isn't actually true. This claim was simply a marketing device created by Kellogg® in the 1800s to sell their cereals.

My best advice for breakfast is to listen to your body. We are each so different. Although your friend might require breakfast to function, you might find you feel sharper and better all-around without it. Just make sure a smaller meal (or no meal) in the morning doesn't equate to overeating later in the day. If you do choose to eat, focus on dietary fat and protein while downplaying the carbohydrate portion.

If you eat a high-carb breakfast, you are likely going to experience a blood sugar high with a compensatory low to follow that results in fatigue, brain fog, and more carb/sugar cravings later in the day. In other words, you'll be on a roller coaster of sugar highs and lows.

A real breakfast for champions might look like the following:

- Have an egg omelet. Add some non-starchy vegetables (like spinach, kale, mushrooms, bell pepper), cheese if tolerated, or maybe even a little uncured bacon.

- If you're in a hurry, eat a few scrambled eggs topped with salsa or some extra virgin olive oil and salt.

- Enjoy some full-fat, plain Greek yogurt with a sprinkling of berries and maybe some nuts and seeds.

- Blend a protein shake that has some kind of dietary fat in it, like cream, coconut milk, MCT oil, or avocado oil. Consider adding a little frozen spinach, a few berries, and ice prior to blending.

Avoid:

- French toast, pancakes, bagels, or waffles topped with fruit.

- Raisin bran (or any hot/cold cereal) with skim milk and a banana.

- Fruit-flavored yogurt topped with granola and fruit.

These breakfasts have very little protein and dietary fat and are laden with sugar, probably around 20 teaspoons' worth in each option. As for beverages, stick with water, tea, or coffee with **real** cream.

Lunches can be difficult. Maybe you go out to lunch for business meetings, or maybe your morning is too hectic to prep a healthy meal. If your breakfast is small or nonexistent, then lunch is going to be an important part of your schedule to ensure that you don't overeat at dinner. If you know your mornings are busy, try to prep your lunch the evening before.

Some good options might be:

- Leftovers from dinner. Perhaps some leftover grilled steak, chicken, fish, or tofu on top of a bowl of greens coated with full fat dressing, cheese, and a few nuts. Add a variety of cut-up veggies if you have time.

- Chicken, firm tofu, or tuna salad. Use avocado -oil-based mayonnaise, which helps to decrease inflammation. Add jicama or turmeric to the mix. Use romaine lettuce leaves instead of bread.

- A burger without the bun and a side salad. (When going out or taking out, you'll find restaurants are pretty accommodating when you ask to substitute veggies in place of the grain.)

Avoid:

- Heavy, greasy carbs. These are hard to digest and will leave you feeling too full and lethargic. Certain food, such as hamburgers with fries; bowls heavy with rice, corn, and beans; and sandwiches with potato chips or an apple, soda, and a cookie, will cause a blood glucose spike with a low to follow, making the 3:00– 5:00 pm slump a huge struggle.

I challenge you to experiment with these suggestions and practice nailing down how you are going to fuel your body for the first half of the day.

At PHD Weight Loss, we make the overcomplicated and daunting task of dropping weight simple, efficient and reliable. We map out a meal plan for you, guiding you on exactly what to eat and when to eat it, in order to drop weight consistently while supporting your metabolism.

During your weekly one-on-one coaching sessions with our nutritionists, dietitians, and life coaches, we review and tweak your meal plan. We educate on nutrition, but knowledge is only potential power, thus we coach you from a behavioral and mental/emotional standpoint, ensuring that we are creating true sustainable change.

The *Reset the Scale Method* is unique. Our protocol does not fit within a specific definition of a "diet." For example, we do not promote a:

- Keto diet.
- Paleo diet.
- Atkins diet.
- High-protein diet.
- High-fat diet.

We don't count calories, points, or anything, for that matter! We don't "subscribe" to a specific diet because we implement a protocol customized to you and your individual carbohydrate tolerance level.

What makes us incredibly unique from a dietary perspective is that we can create a meal plan for anyone with any need. For instance:

- If you have gut issues, we help you learn to overcome them.

- If you're an athlete wanting to optimize performance, we'll get you there.

- If you want to or don't want to eat animal products, we can help do what's best for you.

- If you desire to be in ketosis, we gently guide you in that direction.

- We can successfully accomplish any goal by creating your healthy custom plan!

If this answer doesn't seem thorough enough, I hear you. Some of our clients feel more comfortable comparing a new concept to something familiar. If this is the case for you, you can think of the PHD lifestyle like a modified, sophisticated version of the Mediterranean diet. It's a very effective and efficient dietary approach for successful weight loss recovery.

The *Reset the Scale Method* is a gentle approach that's healthy for ALL your organs and systems:

- It won't put stress on any aspect of your body. It works by reducing inflammation, allowing inflammatory conditions like high blood pressure, gout, and high cholesterol to fall away (and quickly for most people).

- You'll no longer suffer from heartburn or bloating.

- Very likely (and rapidly), your blood pressure and blood sugar will normalize.

- There's no need to take a whole host of supplements because this eating style is nutrient dense.

In addition to changing your diet, being aware of your lifestyle habits is imperative, so I recommend that you consider focusing on two key lifestyle strategies that you can implement right away.

Lifestyle Strategy #1:
SLEEP

If there is one thing you can do for your body, specifically your brain health, it is sleep. Adequate sleep restocks, restores, and prepares your body—it has a huge impact on your immunity as well (Prather et al., 2015).

One recent study looked at amount of sleep and its impact on the number of antibodies made after the flu vaccine after 1 and 4 months. There were significantly less antibodies made with short sleep (defined as less than 4–5 hours a night) (Prather et al., 2020).

There is also a lot of research looking at sleep and weight loss. We see increased hunger and stress hormones along with higher food (specifically carb) intake with short sleep. Additionally, there have been studies looking at groups who slept 7+ hours compared to those who slept less than 7 hours. Despite eating the same amount, the folks who slept less, weighed more (Hanlon et al., 2016; Spiegel et al., 2004).

The most important thing you want to think about when it comes to sleep is going to bed and waking up at the same time every day. There is also a great trick you can use from Craig Ballantyne, author of *The Perfect Day Formula*, called the 10-3-2-1-0 formula. This means 10 hours before bed, no more caffeine; 3 hours before bed, no more food or alcohol; 2 hours before bed, no more work; 1 hour before bed, no more screens; and 0 is the number of times you hit the snooze button in the morning. I encourage you to give it a try!

Lifestyle Strategy #2:
STRESS MANAGEMENT

Whether it's the result of high levels of the stress hormone, cortisol, unhealthy stress-induced behaviors, or a combination of the two, the link between stress and weight gain is glaring and often out of your control. Just as your medical background can have a big impact on your weight loss journey—such as what will work and what won't—so will your stress levels. Even if your diet remains consistent but you're in a high state of stress, the stress alone can cause weight gain.

Let's talk about some steps you can engage in to manage your stress.

1. Get out in nature. Research shows that being outside stimulates your body to release dopamine, the feel-good neurotransmitter (Williams, 2017). So, get outside and soak up your surroundings!

2. Establish a routine for yourself because the brain loves certainty. This means going to sleep and waking at the same time each day and having a schedule for the day that you create the night before. If weight loss is your goal, you need to have a clear, precise and easy-to-follow meal plan.

3. Set your intention for the day through journaling, meditation, gratitude practice, or prayer. Research shows this helps the body's hormones to balance (Ng & Wong, 2013).

4. And lastly, focus your attention on your attitude. Your mood and mindset affect your overall well-being, so make a promise to yourself/make it your responsibility to keep

your attitude and mood positive and optimistic. Turn anxiety into excitement, and focus on what's right rather than what's wrong.

When you combine these lifestyle strategies with this unique dietary approach, you can lose weight without hunger or cravings. I know it sounds too good to be true, so I've included some client experiences for you to read. I also suggest you spend some time reading more client experiences on our homepage at www.myphdweightloss.com as these have been left by real people just like you.

"The people here at PHD have made this journey of weight loss a pleasure. They are here to support you every step of the way. I have gained so much happiness and confidence in myself through this journey. I would highly recommend this program to anyone. It is very worth it."

—PHD Client, Bert

CHANGE YOUR MIND
TO CHANGE YOUR LIFE

Eighty percent of any successful change comes from the mind, and losing weight is no different. Dropping weight and successfully keeping it off, for a many of us, is a perpetual process of letting go— letting go of the excess fat weight that is holding you back along with all of the emotions that are tied to it.

Letting go of anything—old habits, a relationship, that favorite pair of blue jeans—is uncomfortable, even if it's for our own good. The same goes for letting go of excess fat weight. Not only are we saying good riddance to the excess fat weight that has made us sick, tired, and for a lot of us, downright depressed, but we are also letting go of the stories, defenses, and identities that this excess weight has created and reinforced.

For most of us, letting go of this weight also means facing, processing, and ultimately letting go of the emotions that are beneath these stories, which have been our truths for many years, and for some of us, our whole lives. Even though these stories are not useful and are no longer serving us, they are still our stories. Therefore, this exciting letting-go adventure, for most of us, usually involves a grieving process, which is normal. It is sometimes uncomfortable, but normal, nonetheless.

During the weight loss process, our stories or defenses, which may exist only in the unconscious or subconscious, can potentially rear their clever heads, presenting as weight loss blocks, "plateaus" or re-sistance to change. Again, this is normal. Let's expect it but also meet it as an indication of and opportunity to examine and transcend a worn-out belief, story, or paradigm.

That's why I always say that the process of drop-ping weight is 80% mental. The mind-body connec-tion is a powerful one; every thought and belief contains inherent intelligence that can facilitate either a faster letting-go process or a slower one.

To honor the letting-go process—to cultivate one that promotes self-examination and healing—I rec-ommend you maximize the following resources to help you let go in an intentional, healthy, and sup-portive way.

- *Behavior modification is the key to success.* Dropping weight isn't just about what and when you eat. That's definitely a component of it (and oftentimes a complicated one), but how you think and feel about what you're doing is just as important. Be aware that your habits and behaviors, those mental and emotional aspects tied to why you eat, are a large part of the process.

- *Self-care practices are another vital key.* Activities such as a prayer/intention setting, meditation, journaling, or practicing gratitude can be very helpful—a combination would be best!

- *Breathing exercises and self-compassion will help keep you on track.* Take a deep breath and give yourself compassion. If you beat yourself up about the numbers on the scale, your weight loss will stop. It's a fact, and I see this all the time. When you practice self-compassion, weight loss and maintenance success happen with ease.

- *Your energy goes where your focus flows.* If you focus on a plateau or relapse, a stall or regain is likely to manifest. Instead, focus your attention on how simple it is to drop weight and maintain it.

- *If you find yourself with cravings or hunger, eat more dietary fat!* More healthy fats are the ticket to satiety and bouncing you back into nutrition success. Restricting calories or even eating everything in moderation, for a lot of us, results in a constant battle of dropping weight only to regain it and/or unrelenting cravings and hunger.

- *Let go of the shame and guilt.* Remember that weight gain isn't your fault. It has nothing to do with willpower, discipline, or personality. If you struggle with your weight, it's not due to a flaw in personality; instead, it's the product of a dysfunctional metabolic situation.

- *Recognize a relapse and move forward.* The process of dropping weight, for many of us, is a similar process to that of addiction recovery. The truth is that a weight-gain relapse is not the end of the world and only needs to be a brief setback. Weight regain is nothing to be ashamed of; it is simply part of the learning and adjustment process. Find the support and accountability you need to move forward from a relapse. A relapse must be viewed as a learning process; if you are learning, then weight-gain relapses will diminish in frequency and duration over time.

- *Lean on a support team!* The vast majority of us struggle with dropping weight and maintaining it on our own. Remember, statistics show that 95% of diets we do on our own flat out fail. Expecting yourself to make significant and complicated changes on your own is unfair. Instead, seek a support system, accountability partner, or anyone who you can count on to always have your back, guiding you in the direction you want to go.

If you are ready to make a change, recognize that it's then also time for you to let go. You deserve it and can do it if you really want to.

"I'm so thankful that I found PHD Weight Loss! The combination of an easy to follow meal plan, supportive coaches, and nutritional education have taught me how to meet my weight loss goals. It's wonderful to feel healthy, energetic, and in control. PHD is a lifestyle change and I'm happy that I have my coaches' continued support to help me maintain my weight loss. Thank you PHD!"

—PHD Client, Denise

BREAK FOOD ADDICTIONS

Over many years and having worked with thousands of clients, I've come to realize that weight loss is an addiction recovery process for many people. It's different for everyone, but most of us are addicted to food for genetic, hormonal, or metabolic reasons. Therefore, when you decide to drop weight, you must recognize that this is a recovery program designed to last for life.

It is for this reason why, at PHD, we emphasize maintenance support and are known not just for weight loss success but also for helping clients keep it off. It's important to understand that the practice of maintenance never ends.

To support this fact, once PHD clients achieve their optimal weight, they enter into our maintenance program that is free for life with continued weekly to monthly accountability, support, and guidance. No matter how you choose to drop weight, ensure that you have a plan for long-term maintenance support because this is where the work must be done when it comes to breaking food addictions.

During your weight loss, it's imperative to work to remove the love shine from foods and drinks proven to increase weight gain, sickness, inflammation, and pain. Slowly, you must break the ties with the foods you say you love that don't love you back. Through this process you'll learn to take that love and direct it where you truly want it to go—your friends, family, pets, and yourself!

Once you hit your goal weight (I suggest even a month or so before this happens), you must establish a new goal that will keep your mindset in a creative and up-leveling state. If you simply hit that goal and enter into maintenance without another peak to reach, you will slide back down, and relapse will be imminent.

Here's the deal: Breaking addiction is uncomfortable. It's met with a lot of emotions we don't expect to arise and don't want to face. However, I've found that there's *no way out but through!*

Dr. Brooke Feinerman, a psychologist who sits on our PHD Advisory Board, suggests these tips to handle addictive food choices:

- The strongest cravings will most likely occur at the end of the day. Plan for them with a routine that helps you stay on track.

- Make a list of specific high-risk places. Example: a social gathering where it's uncomfortable to say no to specific foods. A list helps you plan for situations and develop creative ways to protect your goals.

- Ask an accountability friend for help when you find yourself struggling in your journey.

- Be aware of negative thoughts because they influence your behaviors.

- Practice self-care. By reducing your stress levels, you're more likely to stick to your goals.

- Seek outside support, and don't expect yourself to go about recovery on your own.

I know I've mentioned this many times, but it's important to remember that the condition you're in is not your fault. This metabolic situation you've been caught up in—the hungry fat mass controlling your hunger, cravings and activity level—affects your brain, thoughts and behavior, leading to a futile cycle of continued weight gain.

Now that you understand the need to fully collapse your hungry fat mass and that the process of dropping weight is an emotional one tied to habits, behaviors, and for some, addiction, it's important to understand what you're likely addicted to!

The most common culprits? Primarily sugar in all its varied forms, especially when mixed with highly processed vegetable oils (polyunsaturated fats).

Let's take a deeper look!

Sugar consumption in the United States has increased from 18 pounds per person, per year in 1800 to over 180 pounds per person, per year in recent estimates. That is an increase approaching 600% over 200 years. What was once a rare delight has become a staple of every part of every meal that we consume in our industrialized world (Taubes, 2016).

Researchers have found that sugar stimulates the human brain using the same reward pathway as known addictive drugs.

In fact, some researchers suggest that the addictive properties of sugar are stronger than that of some of even the strongest addictive illicit substances, such as cocaine (Ahmed et al., 2013; Lenoir et al., 2007).

The food industry has used this knowledge, paired with behavioral tactics, to produce products that are not only poor in nutrition but also specifically designed to be addictive.

Ever wonder why not every chip in a bag of Doritos® has the same amount of sweetness or spice? It's a tactic to drive you to eat another handful in order to find the sweetest or spiciest chip in the bag.

In 1977, the food pyramid, paired with nutrition guidelines from the National Institutes of Health and the American Heart Association, placed blame on dietary fat for the perceived increase in heart disease in the United States. Although limited evidence backed these guidelines at the time, pressure from government agencies and the food industry paved the path for an unprecedented change in the way we eat.

Americans listened and decreased intake of dietary fat in order to prevent heart disease. The food industry responded with products that substituted sugar for dietary fat to maintain taste and replaced saturated fat with trans fats and highly processed vegetable oils to preserve shelf life and texture (Teicholz, 2015).

Grocery stores were then stocked with products that met the recommended dietary guidelines. These products were not only touted as healthy but also designed to keep consumers coming back. Sugar, processed fats, behavioral tactics, and additional ingredients, such as MSG, made these substances irresistible to consumers.

Now, over 40 years later, we have raised two generations of Americans who have been drawn away from natural, local, and seasonal foods all the while becoming addicted to highly processed foods, fast food windows, and sugar in all its varied forms. The result is a society that has become dependent on a dubious industry for its nutrition. During this time, Americans have gotten sicker, fatter, and more desperate for help. Health trends have become more extreme, and nutrition "experts" are everywhere, shouting their opinion about the "right" way to eat.

Those who attempt to make a change in the right direction and drop the processed junk foods most often find improved health. However, the vast majority of these attempts to lose weight fail. Even well-designed nutritional approaches will fail unless the underlying behavioral components are addressed and the hungry fat mass is fully collapsed.

The underlying behavior that fuels lifestyle change failure is this addiction to sugar in all its varied forms (organic, all natural, or not), vegetable oils, and highly refined junk foods and drinks. Many of these foods are masked as healthy.

The next time you reach for something to eat, ask yourself: *Am I hungry? Does my body need this food? How will this food make me stronger? Or is this a result of a craving driven by marketing or a behavior driven by addiction?*

The road to addiction recovery starts with acknowledging the problem and is followed by an intense desire to make a change.

MAINTENANCE FOR LIFE

Losing the weight is one thing, but maintaining it is where most people get caught up. Now, however, you understand the foundation required to set yourself up for the greatest success in maintaining your weight loss. Most people position themselves for weight regain right out of the gate through the methods they use to get there, such as:

- Severe calorie restriction.

- Shots/drops/hormones/surgical approaches.

- No nutrition education. (Or if there is, it's the conventional eat less, move more paradigm.)

- No focus on what foods to eat and what foods to reduce and no discussion as to why.

- No behavioral work (truly the key to real transformation).

- No awareness on the addiction recovery piece.

- And usually, no focus on finding their true Optimal Weight sweet spot while failing to fully collapse their excess fat mass, thus, setting themselves up for a metabolic sand-bagging over the course of a few months.

After reading this book, you understand how these points direct a person toward weight loss failure and future regain, but the final aspect we haven't yet discussed is the importance of weight loss maintenance accountability. You see the real work is done once you hit your Optimal Weight. For this reason, continuous maintenance support is the 5th step in the *Reset the Scale Method.*

At PHD Weight Loss, we recognize the importance of long-term maintenance support, thus, we provide this for free, for life. No matter what route you go to lose weight, please make sure you've got the same level of ongoing encouragement once you hit your Optimal Weight.

I want to take a moment to explain a common sabotaging "maintenance mindset" so that you understand the importance of continued support and effort. You see, oftentimes when people hit "Maintenance," there is much excitement and celebration. (And rightfully so as there has been a huge milestone worked toward and hit!)

However, over time, we think we can go back into old habits and behaviors. We believe we can now tolerate our old junk food and drink "loves," but the reality is that we really cannot. It is over time, with consistent monthly Maintenance Accountability Weigh-Ins, that you will learn the secrets to maintaining Optimal Weight for a lifetime.

It's important that you do not think you will know it all after a series of weeks in any weight loss program. Maintenance is another unique learning process. You need to achieve "mastery in maintenance" for long-term weight loss success. It takes 10–12 months minimum of maintenance practice to allow your new habits and behaviors to become a part of your new "natural" state.

At PHD, we will be YOUR TEAM during your "weekly weight loss phase," and we will be there for you just the same during Monthly Maintenance Recovery.

No matter what methods you follow to drop weight, I want you to understand the reality of what maintenance might be for you. There may be weight gains and binge-relapses, and that is not unusual. Do not feel embarrassed or ashamed if you experience this. It happens, and at PHD, we respect the person who comes back in immediately to recover from a binging episode.

These clients, with us behind them, learn from such situations and recover nicely when they report back in for a weigh-in immediately. It is that individual who when thrown from the horse, picks themselves up, dusts themselves off and gets back in the saddle again, resolved to do it better the next time around. I truly respect these clients, and we handle these exact issues with our clients on a daily basis.

A Successful Maintenance Mindset

Throughout the 12+ years I have been practicing in the field of weight management, I have come to understand both what sabotages maintenance and what supports its long-term success. While I have already shared tactics to watch out for, I also want to share with you what I have found allows for true progress. At some point, I came upon an interesting teaching of the Vedas. It's an ancient body of knowledge where yoga, meditation, and Ayurvedic medicine originate.

These teachings say there's no such thing as good and bad. There is no right and wrong. In the Vedas' teachings, there is only:

- Creation.
- Maintenance.
- Destruction.

If we want nature's support, and we do to achieve an elegant and "flowing" life, we must match our life flow with that of nature. Nature's leading theme is creation and progressive change. Nature is constantly evolving and moving forward, and we live in the middle of the action.

To "maintain," we need to be in the mindset of creation. If we live in continuous growth, maintenance comes in second place; it follows right in line naturally. However, if we settle our mindset in the realm of maintenance, it naturally falls into destruction. In terms of weight management, this is the relapse/regain scenario we don't want.

So, the real question is, "*How do we successfully "maintain" weight loss, and how do we do this not only during "normal" life but also during chaos (which usually throws us off our game)?*

The answer is to always embrace the creation state. Don't remove your foot from the gas pedal. A cruise control mindset equals destruction/regain/re-emergence of bad habits.

During the weight loss phase, you have a clear goal in mind: COLLAPSE the hungry, visceral (belly) fat mass, and reach Optimal Weight. One way to look at the creation, maintenance, destruction concept is in the phrase, "*If you're not growing, you're dying.*" You must continue to create, grow, and establish NEW and exciting goals to sustain your success.

Establish goals that guide you to become stronger. This will help you progress and create. Ask yourself:

- *Who do I want to be?*
- *What's the next level for my health, body, and mind?*
- *Where do I want my health and life to be?*
- *What goals do I need to set and reach for myself in my new, vibrant body?*

Maintenance for life is possible, but it requires energy, focus, support and continued growth. It is the 5th step of the *Reset the Scale Method* because your decision to put in the effort during maintenance is even more important than your decision to lose the weight in the first place.

Now that you understand the *5 Steps to Reset the Scale*, it's time for you to make that all-important decision to step into your own life change. When you do, you are choosing to let go of the old (that has given you what you've got that you no longer want), allowing you to proceed into a future of healthy living. I challenge and encourage you to make the leap. It's exciting and it is so worth it!

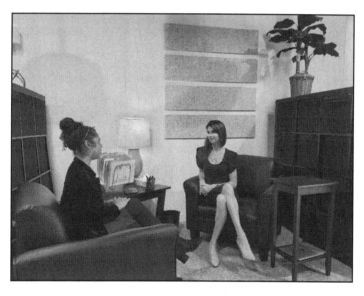

Dr. Lucas consulting with a PHD client.

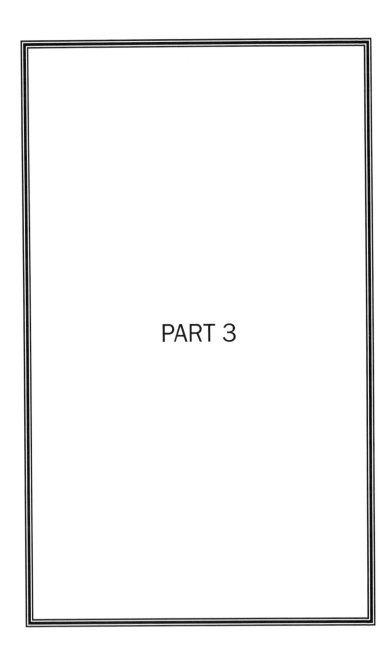

PART 3

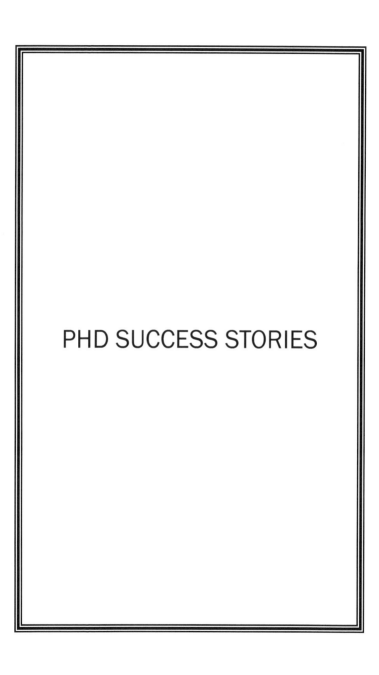

PHD SUCCESS STORIES

"If you follow the program, it works! The support and follow-up are amazing. They will help in any way to assure your success."

—PHD Client, Charmaine

WHAT SOME OF OUR CLIENTS HAVE TO SAY

I thought it would be helpful to share with you several real PHD client experiences. I wanted to highlight not only their experience but also their transformation and elevated mindset resulting from their work with PHD.

These stories are true, and I hope they resonate with you. There are many more client stories on our website for your review as well.

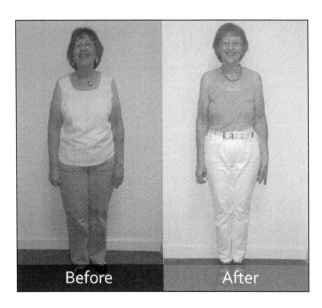

PHD Client, Bobbi (down 45 lbs.)

When people ask me about my PHD Weight Loss experience, my short answer is this: I entered the program for purely cosmetic reasons (i.e., I wanted to lose weight!). I met that goal, and the bonus was that I am healthier than I've ever been in my 70+ years of life.

The brains behind this program is Ashley Lucas, PhD, whose doctorate is in nutrition. This is not a fad diet; there are no gimmicks. It's all science-based and designed to improve your health while reaching your weight loss goal.

Dr. Lucas knows what she's doing. She's smart when it comes to nutrition. She's also very smart when it comes to running a business. She hires the right people; she can't be everywhere at all times. Instead, she trains all of her coaches to be the very best. Dr. Lucas is also the heart and soul of PHD. She cares deeply about all of her clients and employees. The team approach is the perfect way to reach success for everyone.

My journey started after a consultation at PHD. I immediately made the decision to go on the plan and started the next day. Was it a bit scary? You bet it was. But the key to the success of the program is you are never alone; your coaches are with you all the way. Every tool you need is provided.

The backbone of the program is the education piece. Every week when you have the session with your coach, not only is your weight monitored (along with other health data), but there is a also a "lesson" that educates you about all aspects of good health, primarily focusing on food.

You are provided with a handout, so the info shared is reinforced as often as you want to read the materials (I reread mine often). I learned how to read food labels, and that alone has been a key to my success after my initial weight loss. No "diet" plan will work if you don't have the opportunity to learn about the basics of food and how your body processes it.

Also, the daily 30-minute walk, as part of the plan, added to my health journey. My daily walk is part of my routine 3 years later.

I like this analogy that was provided in one of my early coaching sessions: Our bodies love to burn fat for fuel. It is the preferred energy source for almost every cell in our body. Think of fat burn like a propane fireplace: clean, clear, smokeless, and continuous.

Prior to beginning your PHD program, your body likely runs off of carbs/sugar. This is a very easy fuel source for the body to burn, but it is burned so quickly that it leaves the body empty of energy after about 3–4 hours. Think of a sugar/carb metabolism like an old wood burning stove: smokey, sooty, and short-lived. My body has been running like a propane fireplace ever since I completed the PHD program.

Here's a synopsis of my experience: PHD recommended that I lose 30–35 pounds, and they projected it would take 20 weeks to do that. At the end of week 20, I had lost 33 pounds. Then I entered the maintenance phase of the program.

I attended my weekly sessions, continued to lose weight, and switched to biweekly sessions until I had lost another 12 pounds—for a total of a 45-pound weight loss in 10 months. I considered that a success, but I never used the word "stop." I knew how good health felt, and I liked it a lot. I was never going back.

A year later, I had not gained back any of my original weight. As I write this, I am nearing my 3-year "anniversary" of when I started the PHD program. I'm 45 pounds thinner, much healthier, and I'm always happy to share what I have learned with others who are contemplating the same decision I made to join with PHD to improve my life.

—PHD Client, Bobbi

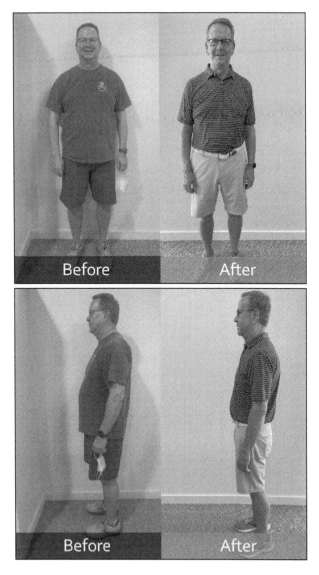

PHD Client, Chris (down 52 lbs.)

I reached out to PHD Weight Loss through the website in early January after hearing a radio commercial on a local sports station. I had a telephone interview the next week and traveled to Greenville, SC, for my initial appointment on January 15th. I had no idea how my life was about to change. And on January 15th, with the help of the Greenville PHD Weight Loss team, I began my journey. I learned that I needed to defeat the visceral fat mass that has sabotaged all of my prior weight loss attempts.

I began the program at 240 pounds. Twice in the last 20 years, I had reached 200 pounds through a diet, not a lifestyle change. At my first weigh-in, my coach, Tara, and I discussed an initial target weight of 185 pounds.

I am not yet at my goal, but I am very close. I have shed a little over 50 pounds, and the transformation in my life is almost indescribable. I feel great physically, and the pain in my knee and ankle is gone. My physician was on board from the start, and after one month, my blood pressure medication was cut in half. After a second month, it was cut in half again, and at the end of three months, I went completely off. Oh what a ride!

—PHD Client, Chris

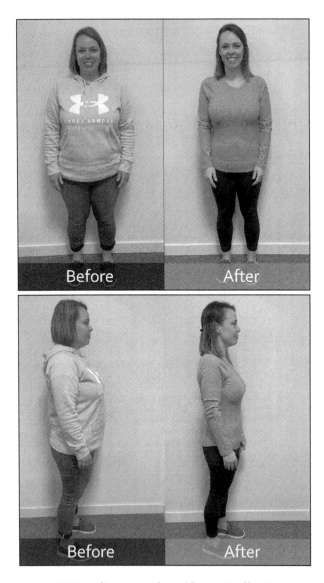

PHD Client, Amber (down 61 lbs.)

Before going to PHD, I had tried to lose weight on my own for several years. I would work out/exercise 5 days a week and lose nothing. I would eat what I thought were "healthy foods" and restrict my diet down to 500-700 calories a day and still not lose any weight. I came to a point where I did not like myself, especially my body and appearance. I hated taking pictures and looking at them. Once I hit 200 lbs., I knew I had to do something. I did not want my teenage daughters to see me struggling mentally, physically or emotionally because I was.

Life now after getting to maintenance is wonderful! I have so much more energy. No low back pain. I can go on hikes without having to stop as often. Exercises that I struggled with in the past, such as sit-ups and squats, I now can do so much easier because my stomach is not in the way!

PHD is amazing. I have learned so much about nutrition throughout this process. I have also learned what healthy foods are and how much better I feel when I eat the right things. The Asheville Team is amazing and will guide you every step of your journey.

—PHD Client, Amber

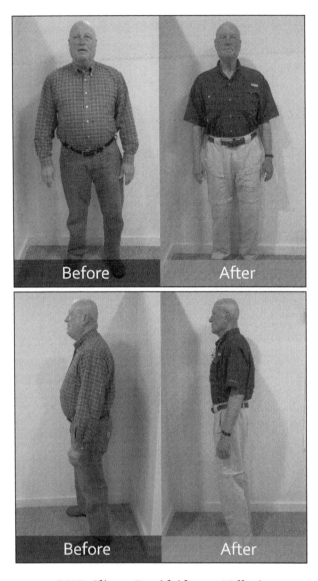

PHD Client, David (down 60 lbs.)

My experience with PHD Weight Loss has been both educational and successful. I have received a tremendous amount of information regarding the nutritional value of food and how to pair foods appropriately.

Armed with this information, I feel confident that I can make healthy choices, not only at the grocery store but also when dining out or dining with friends in their home. My "reach for the stars" goal was 40 pounds.

After five months, under the direction and the encouragement of my coach, Tara, I lost 60 pounds, reduced my body fat by 25% and reduced my metabolic age by 25 years. The entire staff was supportive, always greeting me by name, and I looked forward to my weekly weigh-in and counseling sessions. I left motivated to continue my progress the following week.

Thank you to all the PHD staff, and especially to my coach, Tara, for the inspiration, knowledge and support.

—PHD Client, David

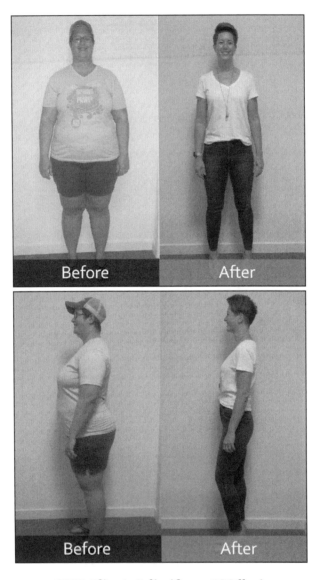

PHD Client, Julie (down 123 lbs.)

My experience with PHD has been a life-saving one, and it's hard to put it in words how grateful I am to this program. A year ago before I found PHD, I was in a place of complacency that I would never be the person I used to be. I'm so glad I had a life-altering moment of fear and desperation and picked up the phone and called PHD (I thought I was on the path to diabetes).

This past year has been so many positive things, not only just losing weight and learning how to listen to my body but also a deeply emotional jour-ney, learning to make better food choices (and preferring those in the long run), understanding how food changes once it's in the body, getting creative in the kitchen (I love to cook so it's been fun creating new recipes), and appreciating the little things that I am no longer self-conscious.

I am in maintenance now officially, and, it is exciting to have hit my goal. But I'm also looking forward to another phase of learning about myself. I think as long as I stay positive, stay kind to myself and listen to my body, I will continue my growth as a person and have success in maintaining this amazing new lifestyle I have found! Thank you PHD. You have given me more than I ever imagined possible; you gave me, ME!

—PHD Client, Julie

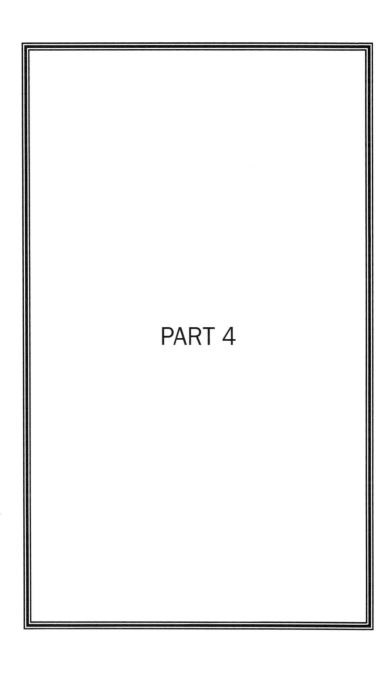

PART 4

THE PATH FORWARD

"PHD helped me find the strength within to over-come my addiction to junk foods. Through their program, I developed amazing techniques for myself. But remember, change starts only when YOU commit to it."

—PHD Client, Trevin

WHO RELIES ON US?

As I mentioned in the beginning of this book, just about any person struggling with weight issues can benefit from working with PHD Weight Loss. It would be our honor to serve you like all the other individuals we have been able to help to date.

Over the last 12 years of practice, I have seen specific groups of individuals lose weight so effectively and in such a sustainable manner that I want to share this with you here to give you a better picture of the types of people we commonly serve. Thousands of these people have relied on us for their weight loss goals and life transformation.

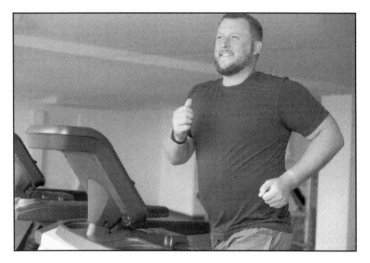

MEN, 45+ YEARS OLD,
WHO WERE ONCE ATHLETES

Why?

As a previous athlete, your body is used to certain ways of eating to support your sport. Usually, you are dealing with a metabolism that has been "burnt" and injuries that keep you from moving the way you used to. The tactics and lifestyle that supported a healthy, fit, active body just don't work anymore and/or just aren't possible at this stage in your life.

Weight loss and behavior change after many years of engrained habits is difficult and confusing, which is why we are here to figure it all out for you and guide you every step of the way. Most of our clients tell us they feel better than they did in their younger years!

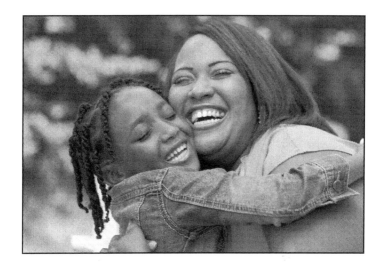

BUSY WOMEN AND MOMS WITH KIDS

Why?

As a busy woman, especially if you've got kids, you just don't have a minute for yourself. Everyone else comes first. You're filled with guilt for even considering doing something for yourself; it doesn't matter if it works. You feel selfish to invest in yourself.

You deserve to have the support needed to find success and to be cared for just like you care for those around you unconditionally. The *Reset the Scale Method* is so simple; the PHD lifestyle is one that supports a busy schedule and every family member no matter their needs. No guilt allowed. It's not selfish to invest in yourself; it's selfish not to.

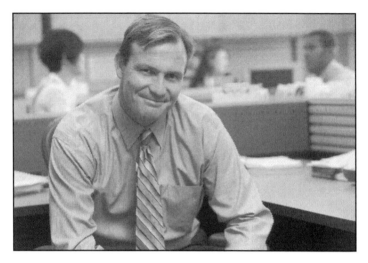

HIGH-PERFORMING BUSINESS PROFESSIONALS AND EXECUTIVES

Why?

As a high-performing business professional, you have no time to waste. You value your time most because you simply don't have an extra minute to give. You have high standards and expect outstanding results. You've *got* to be healthy to do what you do, and you need to look the "part."

I created the *Reset the Scale Method* while sitting in your shoes. PHD is sophisticated, efficient and effective. Bring your A-game, like you do in your career, and you'll experience outstanding, quick, and long-lasting results that will push you to new heights both personally and professionally.

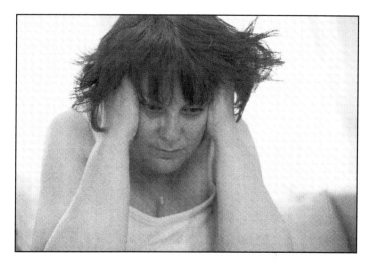

THOSE WHO HAVE TRIED EVERYTHING WITH NO SUCCESS

Why?

If you have tried everything and have been disappointed with your results, understand that you are not a failure. It simply means that you haven't found the right approach to support your needs and body.

If you are stuck in a negative spiral filled with guilt, shame, unworthiness, and emotional eating due to past "failures," please know this within you—there is hope. As difficult as it may be, bring a mindset of optimism and possibility, and you will find a journey that is positive, successful and exciting. PHD will teach you how to trust your body and how to let go both literally and figuratively once and for all!

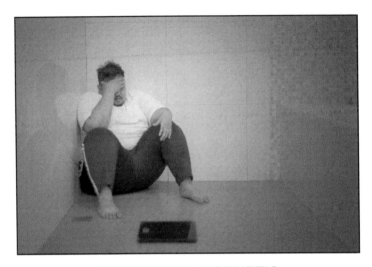

THOSE WITH A GENETIC PREDISPOSITION TOWARD OBESITY

Why?

If you have struggled with your weight since your childhood, you gain weight easily, and/or your parents struggled similarly, it's likely that you have a predisposition to store fat easily.

The good news is that we can help you. Your eating style will be different than what you've been told. Eating less, eating everything in moderation, and moving more aren't the keys to success for you. You need a specific way of eating that supports the uniqueness of your body and long-term accountability for successful maintenance which will ultimately allow for weight loss for life.

THE RESET THE SCALE METHOD
UNIQUE ADVANTAGES

I hope by now that you're convinced that the *Reset the Scale Method* is an effective approach to losing weight once and for all.

You can spend money on all the fad diets, various programs, hormone testing, newest medications, and the hottest supplements. You can even attempt a high -risk surgery, but nothing out there has the all-around positive health impact, sustainable lifestyle, and potential for long-term weight loss success as does this unique approach.

After 15 years of education in the field of nutrition and metabolism, I earned my PhD in sports nutrition and chronic disease and became a licensed, registered dietitian. In 2015, I opened our first brick and mortar PHD Weight Loss office. Five locations later with an expansive nationwide, at-home program, we have helped thousands of people achieve weight loss for life and peak wellness across the nation. We have clients in nearly every state and even serve people who are ready for change internationally.

PHD Weight Loss is so different because we challenge the standard ways of thinking when it comes to weight loss and nutrition. We are not a low-calorie dietary protocol and do not use medications, hormones, injections or supplements.

Our scientific method focuses not only on the metabolic consequences of fat gain but also on the behavioral and psychological aspects, which allows for true behavior change accompanied by efficient fat loss while enhancing skeletal muscle mass percentage.

The PHD dietary approach feels good. You will have no withdrawal symptoms. Hunger and cravings will quickly diminish or become nonexistent when you follow the protocol precisely. You will likely experience enhanced mental clarity, focus and better sleep within the first week! We do this through 4 simple steps:

1. We create your customized meal plan:

During your initial visit, we will create a customized meal plan for you. This plan guides you on what, when and how much to eat as you experience safe, fast and sustainable weight loss. PHD provides 85%

of your food at no additional cost, should you choose to use it. Or we will guide you as you use 100% of your own foods. We provide dining-out guides, take-out guides, grocery shopping lists, everything you need to be successful! We make the process of dropping weight as easy as possible.

2. You receive weekly 1:1 coaching:

Weekly, you will participate in one-on-one coaching, support and accountability sessions with our PHD team nutritionists, dietitians and expert coaches. During these sessions, we review your weekly meal plan, continue to tweak your diet so that you experience continued success, provide nutrition education (unconventional from conventional dietary wisdom), and focus on habit/behavior change to create long-term results.

3. PHD provides a holistic approach with behavioral support:

As mentioned previously, 80% of any life change comes from the mind. We tackle the mental, emotional, habits and behaviors associated with letting go of excess weight. As we discussed in Step #4, we understand that dropping weight for good is an addiction recovery process for many people.

4. You have __FREE maintenance for life__ support:

Letting go of your excess fat weight is one thing, but maintaining it for the long-term requires consistent and continuous support. We understand this, thus, once you achieve your Optimal Weight by dropping the unnecessary fat weight, you are eligible for the best part of PHD, which is our free-for-life maintenance program. We never abandon our clients. You will always be a part of our family. We are your long-term resource and support for all things nutrition and weight-loss related.

As a company, we are upfront, honest and transparent. Once we meet with you in-person or over the phone and learn your story, we will be able to lay out your exact program. During this meeting, we will be able to share with you the length and cost of your care as every program is different, customized to your unique needs. Together, we will establish your Optimal Weight and what is necessary to fully collapse your active fat mass.

There is one last thing to note as you decide if you are ready for change, and that is to realize that up-leveling takes commitment, desire, and determination. You have the power to create change for yourself.

A concept to remember when it comes to doing something in which you might challenge yourself is that you are either going to pay with effort now or pay with regret later.

So, whether you do the work or don't, there is always going to be a price to pay. Success has a cost;

so does failure. You've got to pay your dues no matter what; it's up to you to choose wisely.

If you consider working with PHD, we would be honored to walk by your side in this journey, but please understand that we aren't another fad diet or a $10/month pill that might help you drop the weight in the short term, only to gain it back.

We aren't a membership to a conventional weight loss center; we have no interest in mediocrity or the yo-yo phenomenon. We create dramatic change. We are results-driven and provide a high-quality experience and service that will truly and positively affect every aspect of your life.

So now that you know exactly where we are coming from, who we serve as well as what we do, I want to invite you to take...

"I am 45 lbs. down, my sleep has improved, I have more energy, and I feel better in general. I think the PHD program has had a positive emotional and psychological impact as well. I am more optimistic about many aspects of life than before starting the program. While the weight loss phase was challenging, it was never a burden. Seeing regular results is a great motivator and having great coaching made all the difference. "

—PHD Client, Robert

THE NEXT STEP

Congratulations! You are one step closer to positively impacting your life and dropping this weight once and for all. I hope this book has brought excitement into your life and that you are looking forward to a once in a lifetime opportunity.

Most importantly, I hope that you understand that weight gain isn't your fault. It's not a flaw in your personality but rather a metabolic situation you've been caught up in that you can overcome if you want to. If you've failed in the past, it does not mean that you are a failure. It's because antiquated methodologies have failed you.

It's also important to understand that there is no shame in asking for help. The most successful people out there have coaches. Every top elite athlete in the world wouldn't be able to win a medal without a team of coaches by their side.

Dropping weight with a team of experts behind you is no different. It simply means that you are committed, have an intense desire for change, and are taking action. And as a result of these three things, success is right around the corner.

As you know by now, I am obsessed with challenging the status quo, which ultimately shines through our team, our all-encompassing program, and most importantly, our amazing and committed clients.

Every time I'm in our clinics and have the opportunity to meet with PHD clients, I am overwhelmed with stories of gratitude and hope. They share with me their stories of reversing diabetes, the new confidence they feel when going out with friends, the way their relationship with their spouse has deepened, a desire to date again (!), the way their kids are inspired by their dedication, their newfound desire to get out and explore, and how their physician is awed by their progress, blown away with how their health metrics have done a complete 180.

I love these stories; they put purpose and gratitude in my heart. But you know what? All of this only happens because of them. I always say that it only works if you work it, and that is just what they're doing.

Now it is time for you to decide if you are ready to let go of this weight along with the emotions that are tied to it and break free into an exciting life change.

So, what do you think? Are you ready to transform your body and life? Do you want to be personally guided through your journey of dropping weight allowing the process to be safe, simple, and more certain? Would accountability, unwavering support, and expert knowledge help you bust through barriers and plateaus? Would free maintenance support once you get there help you maintain your recovery?

If you've answered "yes" to any of these questions, PHD Weight Loss and Nutrition might be exactly what you're looking for. The first step is to schedule a 40-minute consultation between you and one of our Certified PHD Consultants. This will give us a chance to "meet" so that we can discuss your specific situation and goals. During this meeting, we will be able to answer all of your questions. At the end of the meeting, you can decide to work with PHD or continue on your own path. There is no obligation, and our goal is to simply guide you on the best path for your specific needs.

To schedule this meeting, please:

Call my offices at: 1-800-674-8991 (Select which option serves you best.)

Remember to mention the code **PHDlife** to receive your consultation at no cost (savings of $25), which is an exclusive bonus for readers of this book.

Prior to your consultation, please visit our website at www.myphdweightloss.com to learn more. Read our client experiences, and study our client before-and-after images to get a good understanding of what to expect.

Lastly, if you found this book inspiring or helpful in any way, please feel free to share it with your friends and family or on social media. If you have any questions, messages, testimonials, or any other encouraging words you would like to share with us, please do so at centraloffice@phdwl.com. We would love to hear from you!

Remember that you can make a change for the rest of your life and simply because you want to.

In health,
Dr. Ashley Lucas

ABOUT DR. ASHLEY LUCAS

Dr. Ashley Lucas is the owner, founder, and advisory consultant for PHD Weight Loss and Nutrition. She has over 15 years of education in the field of nutrition and metabolism and comes to us with a unique background.

Dr. Lucas spent the first 25 years of her life participating in the rigorous training of her professional classical ballet career, constantly devoted to this "passionate pursuit of perfection." However, this deeply rooted "pursuit" was, for her, continuously met with injury and a constant fight with the ballet-specific body type.

As a result, she retired from her professional dancing career, understood the importance nutrition played in her own athletic performance, and started along her path to becoming an expert in the field of nutrition and wellness. Dr. Lucas earned her PhD in Sports Nutrition and Chronic Disease from Virginia Tech and is also a licensed Registered Dietitian.

Her research throughout her 6-year post-graduate doctoral training focused on energy metabolism and the Female Athlete Triad. She was awarded the Academy of Nutrition and Dietetics Scholarship and completed her dietetic internship at The Ohio State University. She passed the national examination registering her as a dietitian offering expert food, wellness, and nutrition services. Dr. Lucas is a nationally renowned speaker, columnist, and leading expert in the field of weight management and behavior change.

While Dr. Lucas began her career in sports nutrition working with athletes nationwide in optimizing performance and body composition, she quickly found a passion in nutrition for obesity-related issues since it was so relevant to her and her family's personal struggles.

After studying literature describing ancestral health and referencing clinical studies dating from current to the early 1800s that successfully treated the (then rare) cases of obesity, in 2015, she developed the PHD Weight Loss approach and established the *Reset the Scale Method*. With a goal of creating a weight loss approach that is successful without medications, fad dieting, severe caloric restriction or chronic levels of exercise, Dr. Lucas designed a program that would work for individuals like her family battling the continuous weight gain seen in today's society.

Dr. Lucas currently lives with her husband and three kids in North Carolina. Together, they embrace growth and opportunities that positively impact others. To learn more about Dr. Lucas, visit www.myphdweightloss.com/the-phd-story. If you're looking for a content-rich, unique speaker on the topic of health and wellness for your in-person or virtual event or podcast, contact her at centraloffice@phdwl.com.

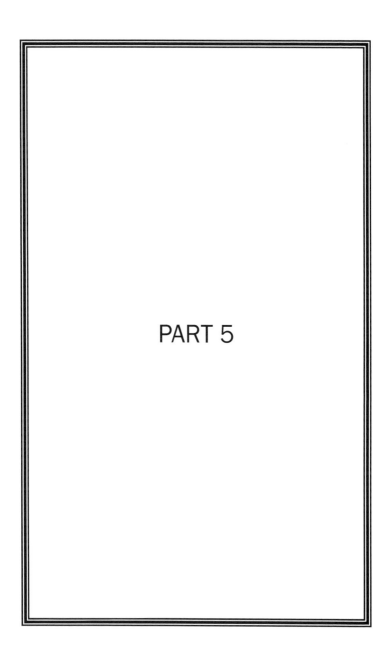

PART 5

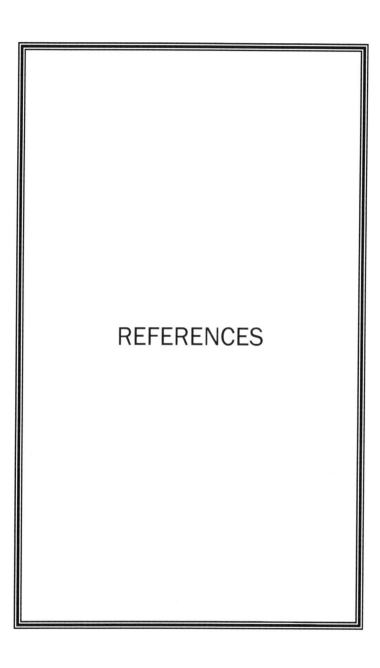

REFERENCES

Ahmed, S. H., Guillem, K., & Vandaele, Y. (2013).
Sugar addiction: pushing the drug-sugar analogy
to the limit. *Current Opinion in Clinical Nutrition
& Metabolic Care*, 16(4), 434-439. https://
doi.org/MCO.0b013e328361c8b8

Ballantyne, C. (2015). *The Perfect Day Formula*. Early to Rise Publishing, LLC.

Bouchard, C., Tremblay, A., Després, J. P., Thériault,
G., Nadeauf, A., Lupien, P. J., … Fournier, G.
(1994). The response to exercise with constant
energy intake in identical twins. *Obesity Research*, 2(5), 400-410. https://doi.org/10.1002/
j.1550-8528.1994.tb00087.x

Hales, C. M., Carroll, M. D., Fryar, C. D., & Ogden, C.
L. (2020, February). *Prevalence of obesity among
adults and youth*: United States, 2017–2018
(NCHS Data Brief). https://www.cdc.gov/nchs/
data/databriefs/db360-h.pdf

Hanlon, E. C., Tasali, E., Leproult, R., Stuhr, K. L.,
Doncheck, E., De Wit, H., … Van Cauter, E.
(2016). Sleep restriction enhances the daily
rhythm of circulating levels of endocannabinoid 2
-arachidonoylglycerol. *Sleep*, 39(3), 653-664.
https://doi.org/10.5665/sleep.5546

Hyman, M. (2016). *Eat Fat, Get Thin: Why the Fat
We Eat Is the Key to Sustained Weight Loss and
Vibrant Health*. Hachette UK.

Johannsen, D. L., Knuth, N. D., Huizenga, R., Rood, J. C., Ravussin, E., & Hall, K. D. (2012). Metabolic slowing with massive weight loss despite preservation of fat-free mass. *The Journal of Clinical Endocrinology & Metabolism*, 97(7), 2489-2496. https://doi.org/10.1210/jc.2012-1444

Keys, A., Brožek, J., Henschel, A., Mickelsen, O., & Taylor, H. L. (1950). *The Biology of Human Starvation*. The University of Minnesota Press.

Lenoir, M., Serre, F., Cantin, L., & Ahmed, S. H. (2007). Intense sweetness surpasses cocaine reward. *PloS one*, 2(8). https://doi.org/10.1371/journal.pone.0000698

Mehta, P., & Fajgenbaum, D. C. (2021). Is severe COVID-19 a cytokine storm syndrome: a hyperinflammatory debate. *Current opinion in rheumatology*, 33(5), 419–430. https://doi.org/10.1097/BOR.0000000000000822

Ng, M. Y., & Wong, W. S. (2013). The differential effects of gratitude and sleep on psychological distress in patients with chronic pain. *Journal of Health Psychology*, 18(2), 263-271. https://doi.org 10.1177/1359105312439733

Prather, A. A., Janicki-Deverts, D., Hall, M. H., & Cohen, S. (2015). Behaviorally assessed sleep and susceptibility to the common cold. *Sleep*, 38(9), 1353-1359. https://doi.org/10.5665/sleep.4968

Prather, A. A., Pressman, S. D., Miller, G. E., & Cohen, S. (2020). Temporal links between self-reported sleep and antibody responses to the influenza vaccine. *International Journal of Behavioral Medicine.* https://doi.org/10.1007/s12529-020-09879-4

Renata Silverio, Daniela Caetano Gonçalves, Márcia Fábia Andrade, Marilia Seelaender, Coronavirus Disease 2019 (COVID-19) and Nutritional Status: The Missing Link?, *Advances in Nutrition*, Volume 12, Issue 3, May 2021, Pages 682–692, https://doi.org/10.1093/advances/nmaa125

Spiegel, K., Leproult, R., L'Hermite-Balériaux, M., Copinschi, G., Penev, P. D., & Van Cauter, E. (2004). Leptin levels are dependent on sleep duration: relationships with sympathovagal balance, carbohydrate regulation, cortisol, and thyrotropin. *The Journal of Clinical Endocrinology & Metabolism*, 89(11), 5762-5771. https://doi.org/10.1210/jc.2004-1003

Taubes, G. (2011). *Why We Get Fat: And What to Do About It.* Alfred A. Knopf.

Taubes, G. (2016). *The Case Against Sugar.* New York. Alfred A. Knopf.

Teicholz, N. (2014). *The Big Fat Surprise: Why Butter, Meat, and Cheese Belong in a Healthy Diet.* Simon & Schuster.

V. Mohamed-Ali, S. Goodrick, A. Rawesh, D. R. Katz, J. M. Miles, J. S. Yudkin, S. Klein, S. W. Coppack, Subcutaneous Adipose Tissue Releases Interleukin-6, But Not Tumor Necrosis Factor-α, in Vivo, *The Journal of Clinical Endocrinology & Metabolism*, Volume 82, Issue 12, 1 December 1997, Pages 4196–4200, https://doi.org/10.1210/jcem.82.12.4450

Volek, J. S., & Phinney, S. D. (2012). *The Art and Science of Low Carbohydrate Performance*. Beyond Obesity LLC.

Williams, F. (2017). *The Nature Fix: Why Nature Makes Us Happier, Healthier, and More Creative*. WW Norton & Company.

Woo, R., Garrow, J. S., & Pi-Sunyer, F. X. (1982). Voluntary food intake during prolonged exercise in obese women. *The American Journal of Clinical Nutrition*, 36(3), 478-484. https://doi.org/10.1093/ajcn/36.3.478

EXCLUSIVE READER RESOURCES

As an exclusive and special gift for readers of *5 Steps to Reset the Scale*, I have created a web page where you can download additional valuable resources, including:

- Bonus trainings from one of our expert PHD coaches on how to tackle stress eating.

- Exclusive interviews with Mike Gallagher and me.

- A video where I show how to read a food label.

- Quick links to 25% off Thorne supplements and free shipping on PHD's favorite electrolytes (only available to PHD clients and readers of this book).

- *And more!*

For Instant Access, Visit:

www.ResetTheScale.com/resources

Made in United States
Orlando, FL
20 September 2022

22606107R00070